Plant-Based Cookbook For Seniors 2023

Enhancing The Plant-Based Lifestyle For Seniors

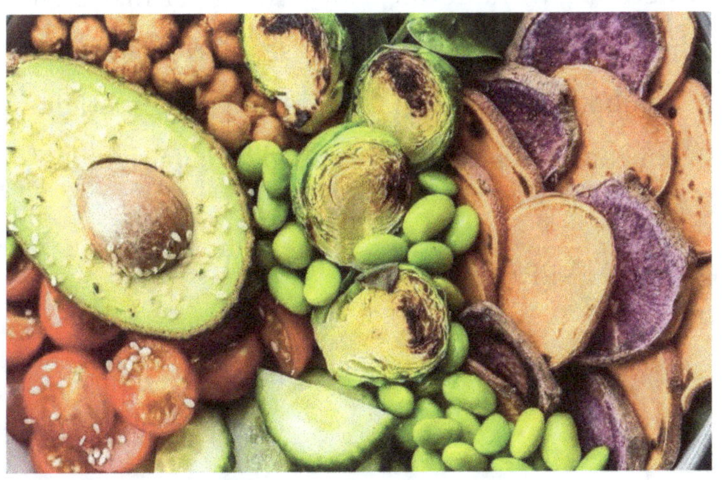

By Debbie Pearl

TABLE OF CONTENTS

WELCOME TO THE PLANT-BASED DIET COOKBOOK FOR SENIORS

I'm happy to have you join us for this memorable occasion as I celebrate the publication of my highly anticipated "Plant-Based Diet Cookbook for Seniors." As I stand before you today and share my personal story and the inspiration for this cookbook, my heart is overflowing with gratitude and love.

I couldn't be more delighted to share this amazing journey with all of you as a fellow senior who has personally experienced the transformational impact of switching to a plant-based diet. This cookbook is more than simply a compilation of dishes; it is a work of love that was created with the goal of preserving our health and vigor as we age.

Please allow me to take you back to the start of my adventure. A few years ago, I discovered that I was dealing with a number of health issues that seemed to affect seniors more often. My energy levels were rapidly declining, and I had trouble keeping my weight within a reasonable range. Chronic illnesses, which often accompany aging, continued to plague my thoughts.

At that point, destiny steered me toward learning more about plant-based diets. Since I had lived my whole life on a typical diet, I was first dubious. But when I learned more about the advantages of a plant-based diet, I was shocked by the mounting scientific evidence for its ability to enhance wellbeing.

My life changed for the better when I switched to a plant-based diet. I saw amazing improvements in both my body and mind. My energy levels increased, my weight stabilized, and I experienced my most vivacious and alive state ever. My connection with food changed from one of simple survival to one of appreciation for the tastes and wonders of nature.

I discovered that there were few resources designed especially for seniors throughout this amazing tour. I ached for a complete cookbook that would provide delicious, nutrient-dense recipes, helpful hints for adjusting, and direction on how to meet our particular nutritional demands.

I set out on a quest to write the "Plant-Based Diet Cookbook for Seniors" because of my enthusiasm and my desire to inspire other elders. This cookbook is the result of in-depth investigation, individual experimentation, and consultation with nutrition specialists. Each recipe is carefully chosen to satisfy our dietary needs and palate preferences.

I'm happy to provide this cookbook to all of you today. It is more than simply a collection of recipes; it is a ray of hope that inspires us to believe in the power of plants and care for our bodies from the inside out. Let's set off on this culinary journey together, enjoying the joys of plant-based cooking and discovering the joy of robust health.

I am very appreciative of the love and support I have received from my family, friends, and the whole team that helped me realize my goal. This project has been created as a result of your support and conviction in it.

I welcome all of the seniors here to go through the cookbook's pages with an open mind and a spirit of exploration. Let the nutrients and tastes of plant-based deliciousness boost you and revitalize your senior years.

I appreciate you being here for such an important day. Here's to living a better and happier life thanks to the benefits of eating plants!

Good appetite!

CHAPTER 1: WHY CHOOSE A PLANT-BASED DIET?

Maintaining excellent health and wellbeing becomes more important as we travel through life and get closer to retirement. Our entire health and quality of life are greatly influenced by the dietary choices we make. The idea of switching to a plant-based diet has drawn more attention recently since it may improve lifespan and health.

A plant-based diet emphasizes eating foods made from plants, such as fruits, vegetables, whole grains, legumes, nuts, and seeds, while reducing or avoiding items made from animals. This eating strategy represents a philosophy that honors the feeding force of nature's wealth rather than just becoming a trend or fad.

Seniors who adopt a plant-based lifestyle may reap a variety of advantages that are tailored to their specific dietary demands and life circumstances. Making the switch to a plant-based diet may be a significant step toward improving health, boosting energy, and living an active and meaningful senior life.

We will examine the strong arguments for older citizens adopting a plant-based diet in this extensive guide. We will examine the benefits of a plant-based diet for seniors, which have been supported by research. These benefits range from the ability to lower the risk of chronic illnesses to maintaining cognitive function, fostering a sustainable future, and more. Additionally, we will address frequent worries, provide helpful advice for adjusting to this way of life, and encourage seniors to confidently begin this life-changing adventure.

This manual's ultimate goal is to enable seniors to make knowledgeable decisions about their nutrition and health by emphasizing the amazing advantages of a plant-based diet in extending life and improving wellbeing. By the completion of this investigation, we anticipate that seniors will have the information and inspiration they need to adopt a plant-based diet as a means of living a longer, healthier, and more fulfilling life. Let's set off on this enlightening adventure together and discover the plethora of benefits that a plant-based diet for seniors can provide.

The Health Benefits of a Plant-Based Diet for Seniors

The significance of maintaining excellent health and wellbeing grows as elders gracefully transition into their golden years. Our bodies change as we age, and we encounter certain health issues. Adopting dietary practices that accommodate our evolving nutritional demands and promote optimum health is essential. A plant-based diet is an appealing option for anybody looking to live a full and active life since it provides a wealth of health advantages that are customized particularly for seniors.

1. Cardiovascular Health: For seniors, a plant-based diet stands out as a heart-healthy choice. Numerous studies have shown the benefits of a plant-based diet, which places a focus on whole grains, fruits, vegetables, and legumes, in lowering cholesterol, lowering the risk of hypertension, and preventing heart disease and stroke. Consuming plant foods that are good for the heart and are high in soluble fiber, antioxidants, and heart-healthy fats helps seniors' cardiovascular risk factors and improves their heart health.

2. Diabetes Management and Prevention: Because insulin sensitivity often decreases with age, seniors are more vulnerable to type 2 diabetes. A plant-based diet, especially one rich in complex carbohydrates and low in processed sugars, may successfully control blood sugar levels and lower the risk of developing diabetes. Plant-based meals include vital nutrients and fiber that help with weight management and improve insulin sensitivity, providing a potential strategy for managing diabetes in seniors.

3. Digestive Health and Regularity: A diet high in fiber from plants helps seniors have great digestive health and regularity. Vegetables, fruits, and whole grains are high in fiber, which promotes regular bowel movements, eases constipation, and keeps the gut healthy. In older people, a healthy digestive tract is important for comfort and general wellbeing.

4. Weight Management and Metabolism: Due to age-related metabolic changes and decreased physical activity, seniors often struggle to maintain a healthy weight. Plant-based diets may help you lose weight since they often include more fiber and fewer calories than conventional diets. The quantity of plant foods that are high in nutrients makes it easier for seniors to feel happy and full, which lowers their risk of overeating and supports a healthy weight.

5. Bone Health and Osteoporosis Prevention: Seniors must consume enough calcium and vitamin D to preserve healthy bones and fend against osteoporosis. The health of your bones may be efficiently supported by calcium-rich plant-based foods including leafy greens, tofu, and fortified plant milks. Additionally, owing to their reduced acid load as compared to animal-based diets, plant-based diets may minimize the risk of bone resorption and fractures.

6. immunological system support: Seniors may see a decline in immunological function as they age, leaving them more prone to infections and diseases. A plant-based diet high in immune-stimulating vitamins and minerals including zinc, vitamin C, and vitamin E may promote general health by enhancing the immunological response. Plant-based meals include antioxidants that are essential for shielding cells from oxidative stress and maintaining a healthy immune system.

7. Anti-Inflammatory Effects: Age-related disorders and chronic inflammation are both major concerns for seniors. The anti-inflammatory benefits of plant-based diets are widely established, with an emphasis on complete, unprocessed foods that help lessen systemic inflammation and enhance general wellbeing.

8. Cognitive performance and Brain Health: As people age, the effects of nutrition on cognitive performance become more obvious. Seniors may retain their cognitive function and memory as they age by eating a plant-based diet high in antioxidants, polyphenols, and omega-3 fatty acids. Consuming a variety of colorful produce, nuts, seeds, and nuts may help to maintain brain function and lower the risk of cognitive decline.

9. Improved Energy and Vitality: Seniors often want more energy and vitality to participate in the activities they like. Diets rich in plant-based nutrients, vitamins, and minerals support an active and vibrant lifestyle by providing sustained energy throughout the day.

10. Managing Menopause and Hormone Balance: Menopause may cause hormonal changes and associated symptoms in older women. The natural phytoestrogens included in a plant-based diet may help regulate hormones, reduce menopausal symptoms, and support hormonal balance.

11. Living a plant-based diet has been linked to longer life expectancy and a lower chance of developing age-related disorders. An abundance of antioxidants and minerals included in plant-based diets boost cellular repair and lessen cellular damage, which helps people age gracefully.

12. Cancer Prevention and Mitigation: While no diet can completely guard against cancer, plant-based diets have shown promise in the management and prevention of the disease. The richness of phytochemicals and antioxidants in plant meals may lower the chance of developing certain cancers and improve the prognosis for cancer patients in their senior years.

13. Psychological Well-Being and Mental Health: As seniors go through life's transformations, mental health is of the utmost significance. Positive mood states and a lower incidence of sadness and anxiety have both been associated with plant-based diets. Enhancing mental health and emotional balance by nourishing the gut-brain link with a plant-based diet is possible.

In conclusion, a plant-based diet has several health advantages that are especially beneficial for older people. Adopting this dietary strategy may benefit immunological support, cognitive function, energy levels, hormonal balance, lifespan, cancer prevention, digestive health, weight control, bone health, cardiovascular health, and emotional well-being. A plant-based diet offers seniors looking to maximize their health and vitality in their senior years an appealing alternative because to its wide variety of minerals, antioxidants, and phytochemicals. The benefits of eating a plant-based diet become even more obvious as we get older, providing a road to a longer, healthier, and more happy senior life.

CHAPTER 2: ESSENTIAL NUTRIENTS FOR SENIOR HEALTH ON A PLANT-BASED DIET

For seniors, a plant-based diet that emphasizes nutritious plant foods including fruits, vegetables, whole grains, legumes, nuts, and seeds has several health advantages. Meeting our bodies' key nutritional demands becomes more and more important as we age because of the many changes our bodies go through. Seniors who live a plant-based diet should make sure they get a variety of essential nutrients to maintain their health and wellbeing. Let's examine the crucial nutrients for aging adults' health on a plant-based diet and the finest sources to include in our meals on a regular basis.

1. **Protein:** Maintaining muscular growth, boosting immune system health, and fostering tissue repair all depend on protein. Despite the fact

that plant-based diets often include less protein than animal-based diets, seniors may still get enough protein from a variety of plant sources. The best plant-based protein sources for seniors include legumes (beans, lentils, chickpeas), tofu, tempeh, edamame, seitan, nuts, seeds, and whole grains.

2. Vitamin B12: The production of red blood cells and proper neurological function both depend on vitamin B12. Since vitamin B12 is predominantly found in animal sources, seniors who eat a plant-based diet must make sure they are getting enough of it. Seniors might include fortified plant milks, cereals, and nutritional yeast in their meals or, if required, think about taking vitamin B12 pills.

3. Omega-3 Fatty Acids: The heart and the brain both depend on omega-3 fatty acids for proper operation. Seniors may get omega-3 fatty acids through plant-based foods including chia seeds, flaxseeds, hemp seeds, walnuts, and supplements made from algae, which are rich in DHA and EPA.

4. Calcium: Calcium is necessary for bone health, particularly in older adults who are more susceptible to osteoporosis. Fortified plant milks (soy, almond, and oat), calcium-fortified tofu, leafy greens (collard, kale, and bok choy), broccoli, and almonds are some examples of calcium-rich plant foods.

5. Vitamin D: Vitamin D helps the body absorb calcium and maintains bone health. Despite the fact that sunshine is a natural source of vitamin D, older people may get less sun exposure, necessitating the use of supplements or fortified foods including cereals, orange juice, and plant milks that are fortified with the vitamin.

6. Iron: Iron is necessary for the blood to deliver oxygen. Lentils, tofu, tempeh, beans, chickpeas, quinoa, pumpkin seeds, fortified cereals, and dried fruits like apricots and raisins are some examples of plant-based sources of iron. Iron absorption is improved when vitamin C-rich foods (such as citrus fruits, bell peppers, and broccoli) are consumed with meals high in iron.

7. Vitamin C: Vitamin C promotes collagen production, wound healing, and the immune system. Oranges, grapefruits, strawberries, kiwis, bell peppers, broccoli, tomatoes, and citrus fruits are good sources of vitamin C for seniors.

8. Zinc: Zinc is crucial for immune system health and wound healing. Legumes, nuts, seeds, whole grains, and cereals with added vitamins and minerals are plant-based sources of zinc.

9. Fiber: Fiber encourages regular bowel motions, improves digestive health, and lowers blood sugar levels. Fruits, vegetables, whole grains, legumes, nuts, and seeds all provide fiber that seniors may consume.

10. Potassium: Potassium is essential for maintaining normal blood pressure and heart health. Potassium may be found in bananas, potatoes, sweet potatoes, spinach, beans, and oranges, among other plant-based foods.

11. Magnesium: Magnesium helps to maintain bone health, muscular function, and energy generation. Nuts, seeds, legumes, leafy greens, whole grains, and avocados are some examples of plant-based sources of magnesium.

12. Antioxidants: Plant-based diets are abundant in antioxidants, which aid in the elimination of free radicals and the reduction of oxidative stress. Antioxidants are abundant in berries, kale, spinach, tomatoes, and carrots, as well as other colorful fruits and vegetables.

13. Vitamin K: Vitamin K is necessary for healthy bone development and blood clotting. Leafy greens, broccoli, and Brussels sprouts are all good sources of vitamin K for seniors.

14. Vitamin E: Vitamin E is an antioxidant that promotes the health of the skin and the immune system. Avocados, almonds, sunflower seeds, spinach, and other plants are good sources of vitamin E.

15. Folate: Folate plays an important role in DNA synthesis and cell division. Beans, leafy greens, lentils, chickpeas, and fortified cereals are a few plant-based sources of folate.

Finally, a plant-based diet may provide seniors a multitude of vital nutrients needed to sustain their health and wellbeing. Seniors may ensure they satisfy their nutritional requirements and take advantage of the numerous health advantages of a plant-based diet by including a range of nutrient-dense plant foods in their regular meals. The best way to maximize nutrient intake and maintain senior health on a plant-based diet is to speak with a certified dietitian or other healthcare expert.

Essential Kitchen Tools And Equipments

Cooking is an art that enriches our lives with happiness, sustenance, and creativity. To prepare scrumptious and healthful plant-based meals, seniors starting a plant-based diet journey need the proper cooking utensils and equipment. These instruments not only make cooking easier, but also more pleasurable and productive. Let's look at the necessary appliances and equipments for the kitchen that seniors may utilize to cook delicious plant-based meals.

1. A superior chef's knife: Any cook, including elders, needs a good, strong chef's knife in the kitchen. Fruits, vegetables, and other plant-based components may be sliced precisely with its versatility. A high-quality chef's knife guarantees safer and more pleasant cutting, lowering the possibility of mishaps.

2. Cutting Board: A sturdy, cleanable cutting board is a need in the kitchen. Choose a cutting board made of bamboo or high-density polyethylene since they are kind to knife blades and provide a sanitary work surface.

3. Vegetable Peeler: Peeling fruits and vegetables is a cinch with a sturdy vegetable peeler. Seniors who like to peel specific fruits and vegetables for improved digestion or personal taste may find it especially helpful.

4. Blender or food processor: Seniors may use a blender or food processor to make purees, sauces, dips, and smoothies from a variety of plant-based products. Seniors may enjoy a variety of textures and tastes in their food thanks to these tools that make meal preparation easier.

5. Immersion Blender: Also referred to as a hand blender, an immersion blender is a useful appliance for mixing soups and sauces in the pot itself without the need to transfer them to another blender. It is appropriate for seniors with limited mobility or strength since it is lightweight and simple to wield.

6. Salad spinner: A salad spinner is great for seniors who want to eat healthy salads with colorful, crisp greens. By effectively draining extra water from cleaned lettuce and greens, this gadget makes sure salads are beautifully crisp and ready to eat.

7. Steamer Basket: Keeping the nutrients and tastes of veggies while gently cooking them requires the use of a steamer basket. Vegetables like broccoli, cauliflower, carrots, and green beans may be perfectly steamed by seniors without much difficulty.

8. Non-Stick Cookware: Seniors benefit greatly from non-stick cookware since it uses less oil while cooking, allowing for the simpler preparation of healthy plant-based meals. The trouble of washing after cooking is also reduced by the simplicity of cleaning these cookware alternatives.

9. An oven or toaster oven is necessary for baking delicious plant-based foods including roasted vegetables, casseroles, and desserts. Seniors may dabble with baking without requiring a full-size oven thanks to this.

10. Slow Cooker or Crock-Pot: Seniors may easily produce delectable stews, soups, and one-pot meals with the help of this time- and energy-saving equipment. It is perfect for elders who want cooking that they can set and forget.

11. Measuring Cups and Spoons: Accurate measures are essential in cooking, particularly for seniors who follow recipes that call for plants. A set of measuring spoons and cups is an investment that guarantees precise ingredient proportions for mouthwatering outcomes.

12. Colander: A colander may be used to drain and rinse food items including pasta, beans, lentils, quinoa, and other grains. It may be used by seniors to drain extra water from cooked grains or to wash produce before eating.

13. Baking sheets and pans are necessary for baking baked items like cookies, muffins, and bread as well as for roasting vegetables. For simpler cleaning, use items that are silicone- or non-stick-coated.

14. Herb and Spice Grinder: Seniors may add freshly ground herbs and spices to their plant-based foods to enhance the taste. To easily generate fragrant mixes that give their culinary creations depth, use a herb and spice grinder.

15. Reusable food storage containers: Seniors may easily store leftovers and prepared meals in reusable food storage containers, helping to prevent food waste and encourage systematic meal preparation.

16. Adjustable Mandoline Slicer: An adjustable mandoline slicer enables elders to slice produce precisely and uniformly for reliable cooking outcomes.

17. Whisk: An effective tool for seniors to mix and combine ingredients in batters, dressings, and sauces is a whisk.

18. Citrus Juicer: Seniors can easily add citrus tastes to their foods thanks to a citrus juicer, which makes the process of squeezing fresh juice from lemons, limes, and oranges simple.

19. Using a vegetable spiralizer, senior citizens may become creative with vegetable noodles. This device turns vegetables like carrots, zucchini, and other vegetables into tasty and healthy substitutes for noodles.

20. Silicone Spatulas: Silicone spatulas can effectively scrape the edges of bowls and pans while being kind on non-stick cookware, ensuring that seniors devour every last piece of their plant-based dishes.

In conclusion, having the proper cooking utensils and supplies is crucial for seniors starting their plant-based diet journey. These appliances simplify food preparation, provide user-friendliness, and encourage culinary innovation. Seniors may improve their culinary experience and general pleasure of a plant-based diet by stocking their kitchens with high-quality necessities to make healthful, tasty, and engaging plant-based cuisine.

CHAPTER 3: GUIDELINES FOR GROCERY SHOPPING AND MEAL PLANNING FOR SENIORS

A healthy and balanced plant-based diet requires careful planning of meals and regular supermarket shopping. These procedures not only save time and money, but also guarantee that wholesome meals are accessible every day of the week. The following advice can help you simplify meal planning and grocery shopping, regardless of your experience level with plant-based eating:

1. Establish a Weekly Routine for Meal Planning: Every week, set aside a designated day to arrange your meals. Consider your schedule, dietary needs, and any upcoming social engagements that may have an influence on your meal choices. A weekly schedule keeps you organized and makes sure you eat a variety of healthy meals throughout the week.

2. Make a food Plan: List your food ideas for each day of the week in a meal plan or in a straightforward notebook. Include snacks, lunch, supper, and morning. Make space in your schedule for leftovers and unplanned food attempts.

3. Use Resources for Vegetarian Recipes: For ideas, peruse websites, books, and apps that provide plant-based recipes. To include them in your meal plan, save your favorite recipes. To make the most of seasonal products and fresh vegetables, look for recipes that employ them.

4. Create Balanced Meals: Make sure each meal is balanced by including a range of foods in terms of their colors, nutrients, and macronutrients. To make healthful and filling meals, combine whole grains with a variety of vegetables, fruits, legumes, nuts, and seeds.

5. Prepare some meals in advance for convenience if at all feasible. To save time during the hectic weekdays, prepare cereals, chop veggies, and soak beans and lentils in advance. You may enjoy homemade meals with little effort if you prepare ahead of time and cut down on cooking time.

6. Create a Detailed Grocery List: Based on your meal plan, make a comprehensive grocery list. To facilitate buying, categorize the list into sections for fruits, vegetables, grains, and pantry essentials.

7. Focus on the Outside of the Store: In the grocery store, look for fresh vegetables, whole grains, and plant-based proteins on the outside of the store. Purchases of processed and packaged foods, which are often heavy in added sugars, salt, and artificial additives, should be kept to a minimum.

8. Buy Seasonal and Local food: When feasible, choose food that is in season and that was grown locally. This not only helps local farmers, but seasonal fruit is usually more tasty and fresh.

9. Carefully check Labels: When buying packaged items, check labels carefully. Find items with little additives and easily identified, basic components. Pick foods that are low in harmful fats, salt, and added sugars.

10. Keep Staples on Hand: Keep plant-based staples like whole grains (rice, quinoa, oats), legumes (beans, lentils), nuts, seeds, canned tomatoes, and vegetable broth on hand in your pantry. You can make fast and wholesome dinners if you have these ingredients on hand.

11. Purchase in Bulk: Buying some foods, such as grains, nuts, and seeds, in bulk may save money and cut down on waste from superfluous packaging.

12. Be Conscious of Portion proportions: To reduce waste, take portion proportions into account when purchasing fresh vegetables. Choose smaller servings or think about frozen choices if you don't eat huge amounts of a certain fruit or vegetable.

13. Select Eco-Friendly Options: To minimize plastic waste, use reusable shopping bags. Buy things with little packaging or choose those with environmentally friendly packaging.

14. Adhere to Your Grocery List: By adhering to your grocery list, you may prevent impulsive purchases. Before adding new, alluring items to your shopping basket, see whether your meal plan and dietary objectives are compatible with them.

15. Shop while You're Full: Making impulsive, unhealthy food selections while you're hungry might result. Before you go shopping, have a little snack to help you think things through.

16. Keep Your Home Organized: After going food shopping, arrange your kitchen and refrigerator so that you can quickly find goods. Perishable food should be properly labeled and stored to prevent deterioration.

17. Observe safe food handling and storage procedures to avoid foodborne infections. Pay close attention to the dates on items and consume them within the suggested time ranges.

18. Reduce food waste by repurposing leftovers and freezing parts for later meals. Plan your meals to combine components from different recipes, which will cut down on food waste.

19. Include the Family: If you are preparing food for a family, include them in the meal preparation process. Encourage kids to explore new plant-based dishes by asking for their feedback on the meals they should eat.

20. Be Adventurous and Enjoy the Process: Enjoy trying new foods and dishes as you embark on the journey of a plant-based diet. As you learn the benefits of supporting your body with a plant-based diet, meal planning and grocery shopping can be joyful and fulfilling.

In conclusion, organizing your meals and doing your grocery shopping are crucial habits to keep up with a good plant-based diet. Seniors may enjoy a wide variety of nutrient-dense plant-based meals by preparing a weekly meal plan, a well-organized grocery list, and shopping with awareness. These behaviors encourage not just a healthy and happy lifestyle but also one that is sustainable and fun. Be open to trying new foods, be creative in the kitchen, and enjoy the health advantages of feeding your body nutritious, plant-based foods.

CHAPTER 4: DELICIOUS AND NUTRITIOUS PLANT-BASED BREAKFAST RECIPES FOR SENIORS

A healthy start to the day is provided for seniors by breakfast, which is often regarded as the most significant meal of the day. Accepting a plant-based diet opens the door to a world of mouthwatering, nutrient-rich breakfast alternatives that may promote elder health and energy levels all day long. Let's investigate a number of delicious plant-based breakfast dishes that are also nutrient-dense to help seniors start the day off energetically.

1. Energizing Smoothie Bowl: To make a creamy and nutrient-rich smoothie, combine frozen mixed berries, spinach, banana, almond milk, and a scoop of plant-based protein powder. Sliced fruits, such as strawberries and kiwis, as well as granola, chia seeds, and almond flakes may be added to the smoothie after it has been poured into a bowl.

2. Filling Oatmeal with Nut Butter and Berries: Blend steel-cut oats with water and almond milk until creamy. For extra richness and protein, mix with a teaspoon of almond or peanut butter. Add a few fresh berries, banana slices, and a drizzle of maple syrup or agave nectar to the oats for natural sweetness.

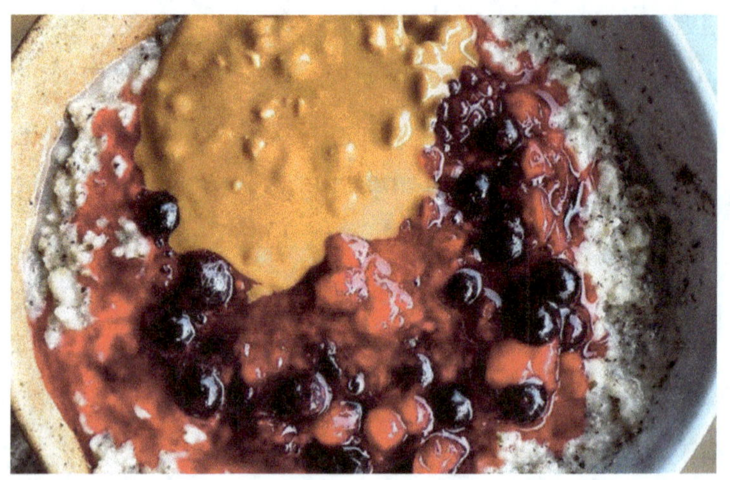

3. Filling Chia Seed Pudding: Combine chia seeds with almond milk, a pinch of vanilla, and a drizzle of maple syrup. For a creamy pudding texture, refrigerate overnight. For a delicious and revitalizing breakfast, top the chia seed pudding with fresh fruit in the morning, such as mango, pineapple, and pomegranate seeds.

4. Protein-Rich Tofu Scramble: Sauté cubed tofu with onions, bell peppers, and spinach in a nonstick skillet with a splash of turmeric and nutritional yeast for a cheesy taste. For a delicious and protein-rich breakfast, serve the tofu scramble with a side of avocado slices and whole-grain bread.

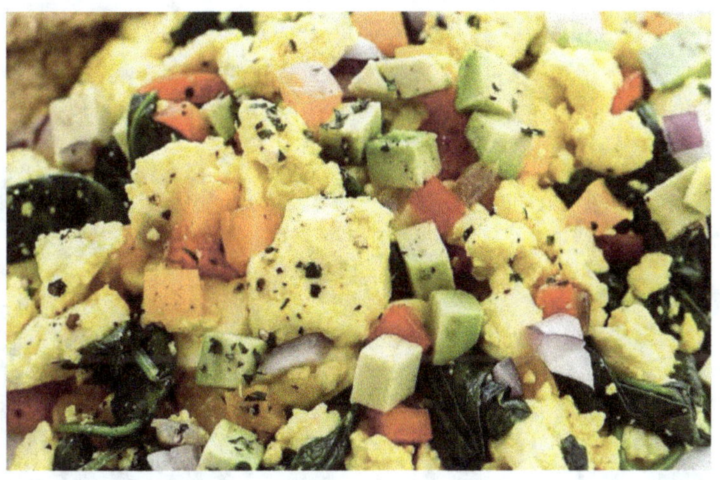

5. Filling Banana Walnut Pancakes: To make the batter for the pancakes, combine mashed ripe bananas with oat flour, almond milk, chopped walnuts, and a dash of cinnamon. In a nonstick skillet, cook the pancakes until golden brown. Garnish with fresh berries and pure maple syrup.

6. Nutty Overnight Oats: To make a jar of nut-flavored overnight oats, combine rolled oats, almond milk, chia seeds, finely chopped almonds, and a little amount of almond butter. For a quick and filling grab-and-go breakfast in the morning, let it rest in the refrigerator overnight.

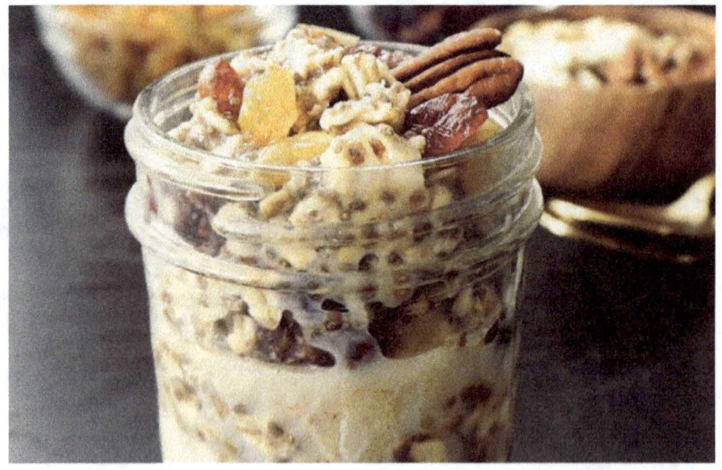

7. Savory Avocado Toast: Mash ripe avocados with a touch of lemon and some salt. Add sliced tomatoes, red onion, and black pepper to the whole-grain bread after spreading the avocado mixture on it. This simple yet filling meal offers taste and good fats.

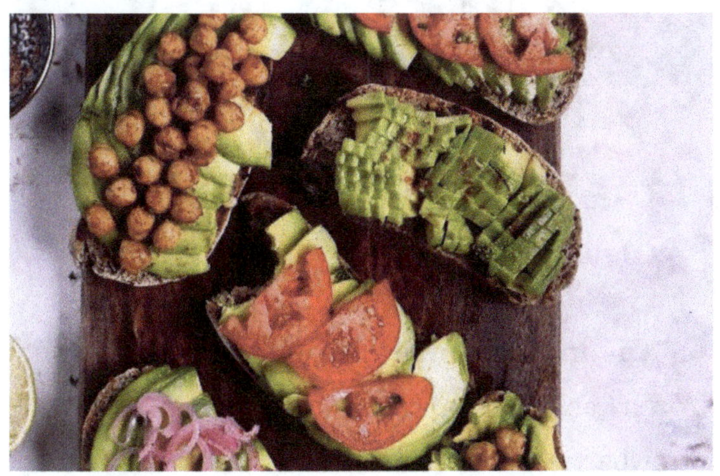

8. Protein-Packed Breakfast Burrito: Add sliced avocado, chopped tomatoes, black beans, scrambled tofu, and spicy sauce to a whole-wheat tortilla. Seniors on the move will love this hearty, protein-packed breakfast burrito that you can wrap up.

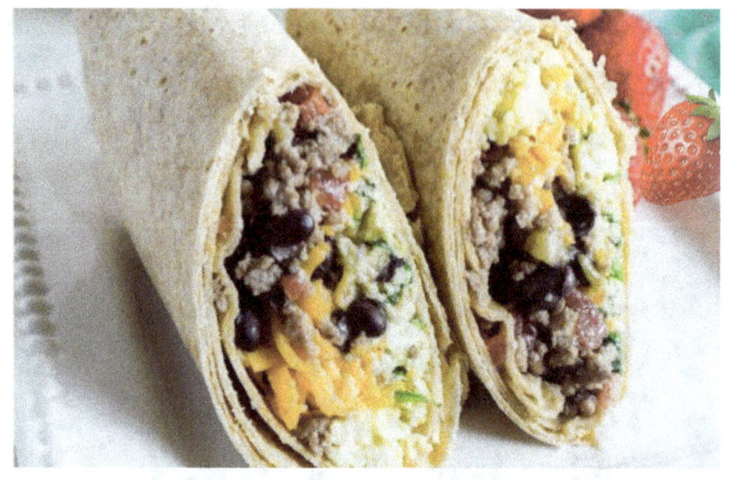

9. An antioxidant-rich acai bowl made with frozen acai puree, banana, and almond milk. Strawberries, blueberries, and kiwis are cut and placed on top of the acai mixture in a bowl. A colorful and wholesome breakfast may be made by adding some granola, coconut flakes, and honey.

10. Spicy Lemon Poppy Seed Muffins: To make these muffins, combine whole wheat flour, almond milk, maple syrup, and lemon zest. These delectable muffins provide a lovely and portable breakfast alternative that are ideal for savoring with a glass of herbal tea or a container of plant-based yogurt.

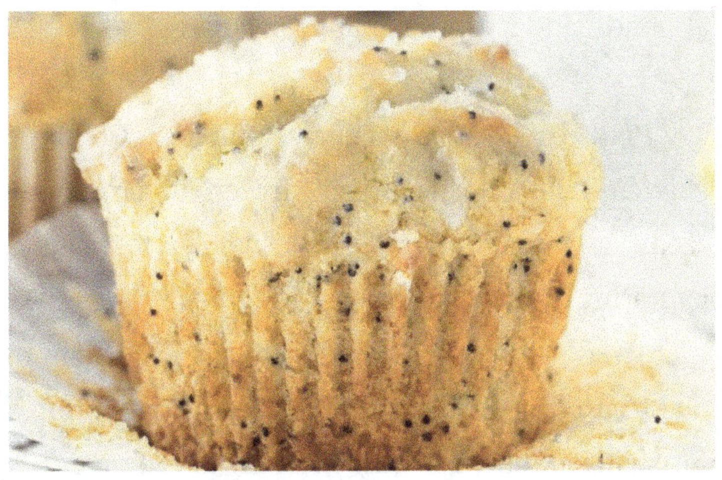

11. Creamy Coconut Chia Pudding: Blend together chia seeds, coconut milk, and a little vanilla flavor. Keep it chilled until it becomes creamy and thick. A tropical-inspired morning treat may be made by topping the coconut chia pudding with mango slices, toasted coconut flakes, and chopped pistachios.

12. Seasonal fruit parfaits, such as berries, peaches, and kiwis, are layered with plant-based yogurt. For a delicious and aesthetically pleasing parfait, add a tablespoon of granola, a scattering of almonds, and a drizzle of honey or agave.

13. Protein-Packed Green Smoothie: Combine kale or spinach, cucumber, frozen banana, chia seeds, and almond milk in a blender to make a hydrating and wholesome green smoothie. Increased protein content with the inclusion of plant-based protein powder makes the smoothie a satisfying and invigorating morning alternative.

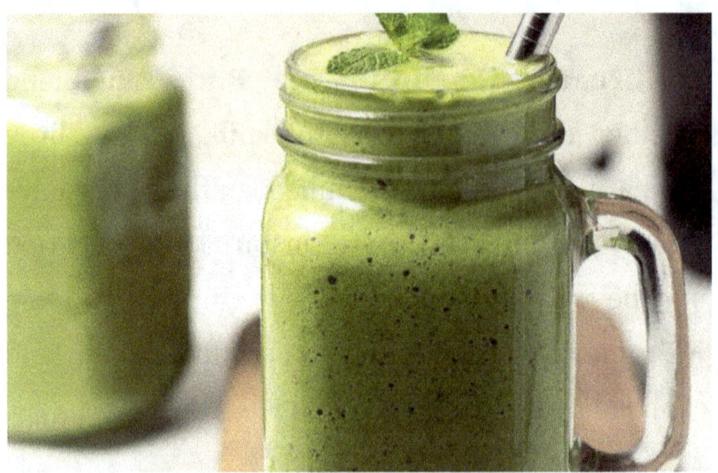

14. Veggie Frittata Cups: Combine a variety of chopped veggies, including bell peppers, zucchini, and cherry tomatoes, with chickpea flour, water, turmeric, nutritional yeast, and other seasonings. For a hearty and filling frittata cup breakfast, pour the mixture into muffin tins and bake until golden.

15. Nut butter and banana sandwich: Spread peanut or almond butter on whole-grain bread and top with slices of banana. Fold the bread to make a tasty, convenient, filling, and nutrient-dense nut butter and banana sandwich.

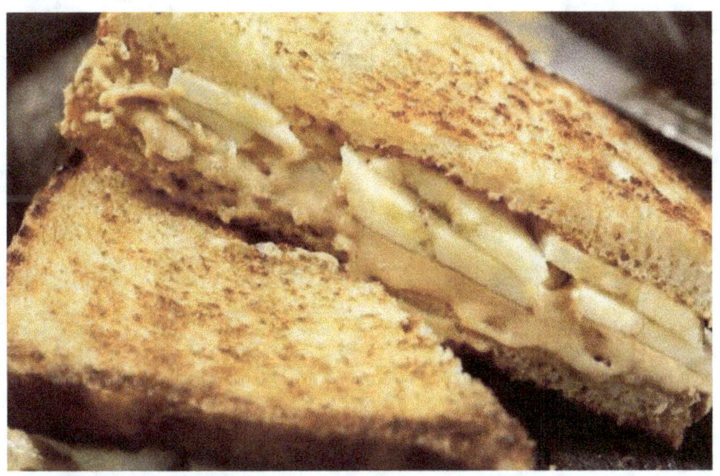

Finally, a plant-based diet provides a variety of scrumptious and nourishing breakfast alternatives for seniors. The important vitamins, minerals, and fiber in these breakfast dishes for seniors' health and wellbeing come from a range of nutrient-dense plant foods. Seniors may enjoy the pleasures and advantages of a plant-based diet while beginning their days with vigor and energy by eating things like smoothie bowls, oatmeal, tofu scramble, or chia seed pudding. Seniors may enjoy breakfast time as they begin a healthy and rewarding plant-based diet by using creativity and the plethora of plant-based products.

CHAPTER 5: WHOLESOME LUNCH IDEAS FOR SENIORS ON A PLANT-BASED DIET

Seniors who love lunch have the chance to have a filling and healthy meal that will keep their bodies going throughout the remainder of the day. A plant-based diet offers a wide variety of scrumptious and healthy lunch alternatives that are packed with nutrients that promote senior health and wellbeing. Investigate a number of plant-based lunch suggestions that are not only filling but also bursting with flavors and textures that seniors will like.

1. Bright Mediterranean Salad: Make a colorful Mediterranean salad by combining cherry tomatoes, cucumbers, bell peppers, red onions, Kalamata olives, and chickpeas. Lunch may be made with a salad that has been dressed with a lemon-tahini dressing, fresh parsley, and a dash of oregano.

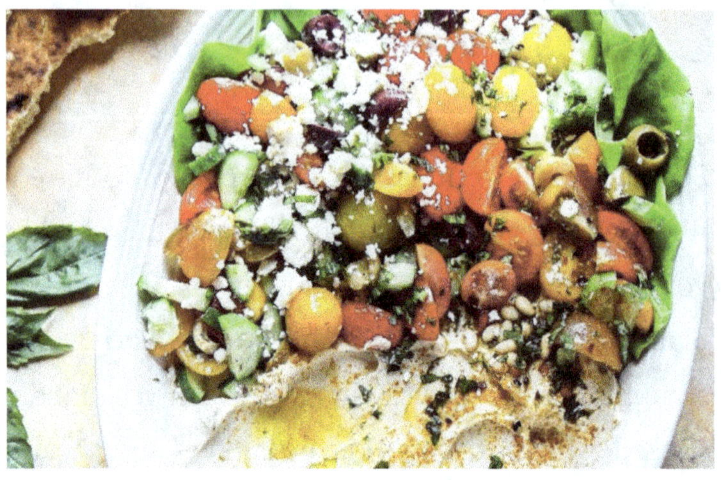

2. Hearty Lentil Soup: Combine green or brown lentils, chopped tomatoes, carrots, celery, and onions to make a warming lentil soup. Add a bay leaf, garlic, and thyme to the soup's seasonings. For a satisfying and healthy lunch, serve the soup with a side of crusty whole-grain bread.

3. Veggie Sushi Rolls: Use nori sheets to roll up a variety of fresh vegetables, such as avocado, cucumber, carrot, and bell pepper, with seasoned sushi rice. An enjoyable and filling plant-based sushi meal may be made by slicing the sushi rolls into bite-sized pieces and serving them with soy sauce, pickled ginger, and wasabi.

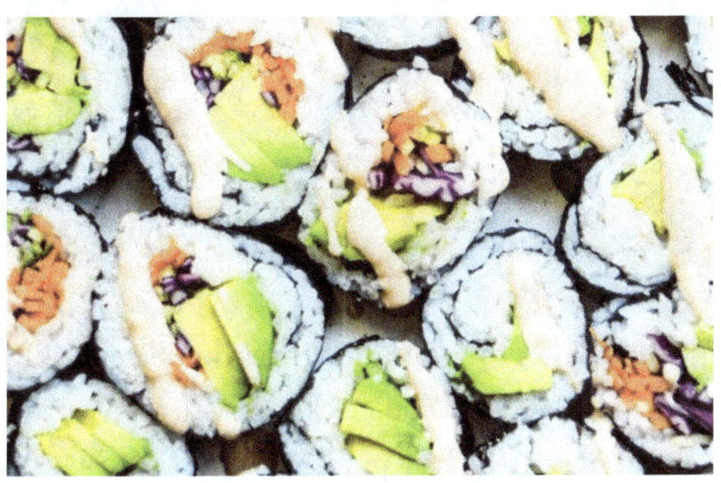

4. Buddha Bowl with Quinoa and Roasted Veggies: Make a Buddha bowl by layering roasted veggies like sweet potatoes, broccoli, and Brussels sprouts on top of a cooked quinoa foundation. For a filling and aesthetically pleasing lunch, include a scoop of hummus, a plateful of greens, and some pumpkin seeds.

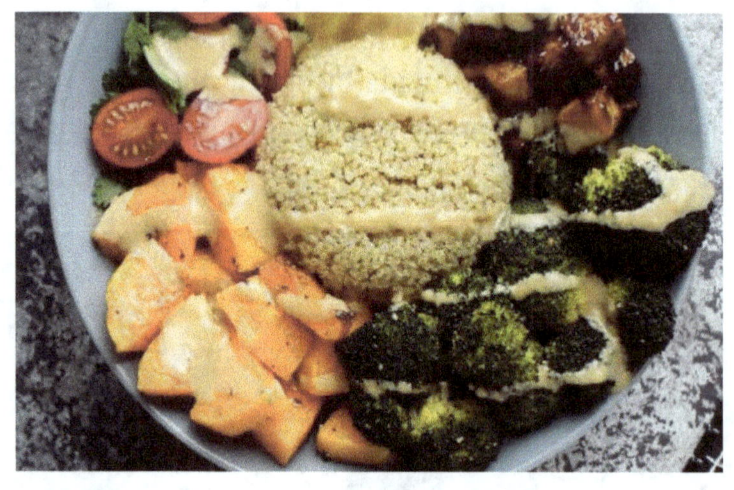

5. Creamy Avocado and Chickpea Sandwich:
Blend ripe avocado and chickpeas with a squeeze of lemon, some minced garlic, and a dash of salt. Spread the smooth avocado-chickpea mixture on whole-grain bread, top it with slices of tomato, cucumber, and sprouts, and you've got yourself a full and tasty sandwich.

6. Quinoa and bean stuffed bell peppers:
Stuff half bell peppers with a mixture of cooked quinoa, black beans, corn, chopped tomatoes, and seasonings. To make the stuffed peppers into a

filling and healthy meal, bake them in the oven until they are soft.

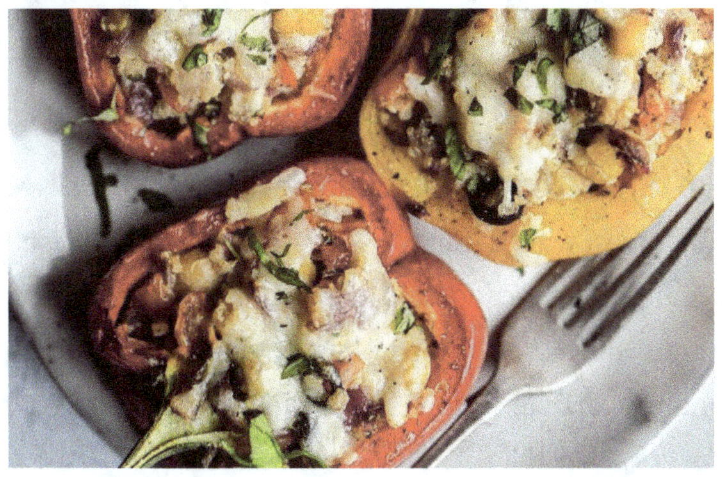

7. Sauté sliced mushrooms, onions, and garlic in a little soy sauce in a nonstick skillet for the spinach and mushroom stir-fry. Cook until wilted after adding new spinach. For an easy and tasty lunch alternative, put the spinach and mushroom stir-fry on top of some brown rice or noodles.

8. Hummus Veggie Wrap: Spread a liberal quantity of hummus on a whole-wheat tortilla and top it with bell pepper slices, baby spinach, and carrots that have been thinly sliced. For an easy-to-grab lunch on the run, roll up the wrap and cut it into pinwheels.

9. Stuffed Sweet Potatoes: Fill baked sweet potatoes with a mixture of black beans, chopped tomatoes, avocado, and cilantro after baking them until they are cooked. For a vibrant and filling lunch, drizzle some lime juice and plant-based yogurt over the packed sweet potatoes.

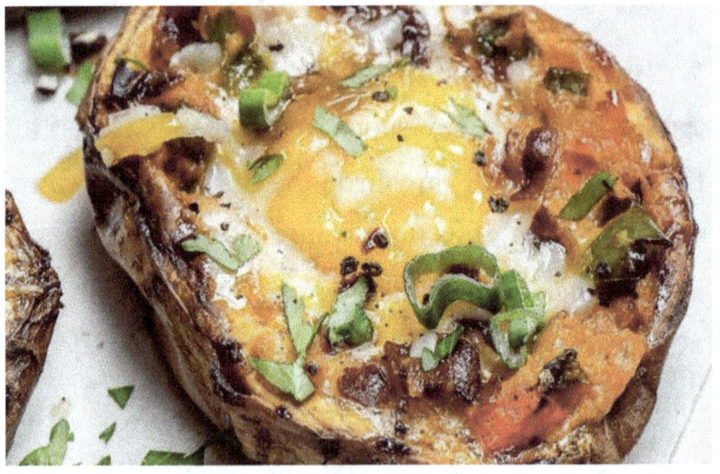

10. Spiralized Zucchini Noodles with Basil Pesto: Combine spiralized zucchini into noodles with a homemade basil pesto prepared from pine nuts, garlic, lemon juice, and nutritional yeast. For a tasty and light lunch, add cherry tomatoes and toasted pine nuts.

11. Curried Chickpea Salad: Combine chopped celery, red onion, and dried cranberries with chickpeas in a curry tahini dressing. For a tasty and protein-rich lunch, place the curried chickpea salad in a whole-grain pita or over a bed of mixed greens.

12. To make the Tomato Basil Bruschetta, dice ripe tomatoes and combine them with fresh basil, chopped garlic, balsamic vinegar, and a splash of olive oil. For a cool and healthy lunch alternative, spread the tomato basil mixture over toast made from whole grain bread.

13. Soba Noodle Salad with Peanut Dressing: Toss cooked soba noodles with shredded carrots, cucumber slices, edamame, and a creamy peanut dressing prepared from peanut butter, soy sauce, lime juice, and a little maple syrup for a filling and tasty lunch.

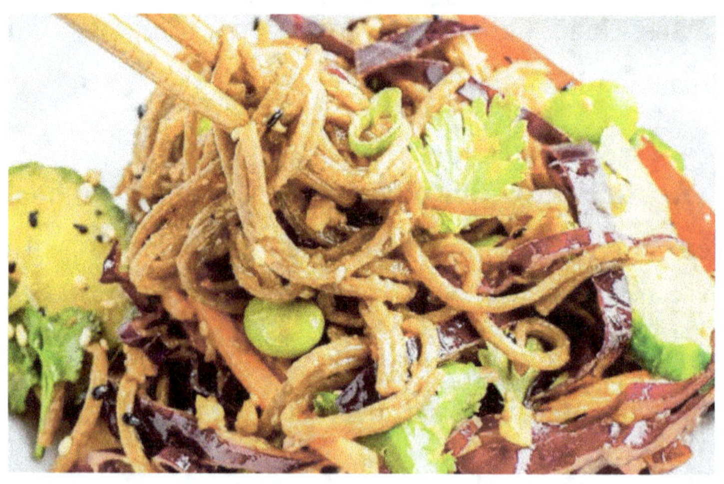

14. Vegetable fajita bowl: Sauté a mixture of bell peppers, onions, and zucchini with fajita spice until soft. For a delicious and healthful lunch, place the vegetable fajita mixture over a bed of cilantro-lime rice and garnish with sliced avocado, salsa, and fresh cilantro.

15. Protein-Rich Tofu Salad: Soak cubed tofu in a combination of ginger, garlic, and soy sauce. Serve the tofu over a salad with mixed greens, cherry tomatoes, cucumber, and a sesame-ginger dressing for a satisfying and protein-rich lunch after gently browning it in the skillet.

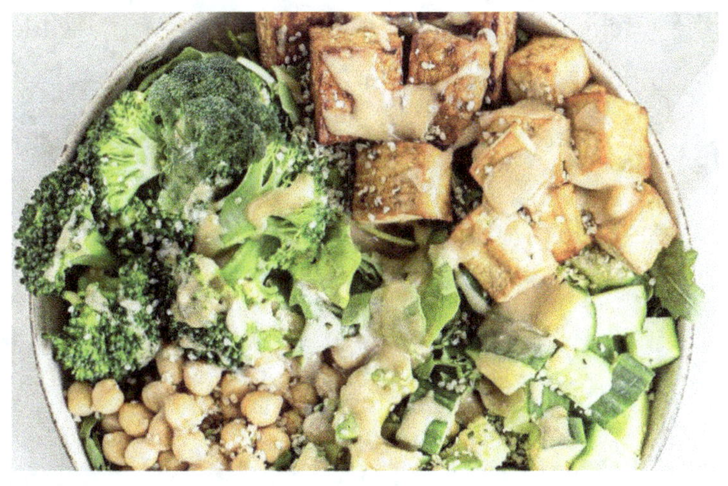

Finally, there are a variety of healthy and scrumptious lunch options available for seniors following a plant-based diet. These plant-based lunch alternatives include a variety of nutrient-rich fruits, vegetables, legumes, and whole grains to provide older citizens necessary vitamins, minerals, fiber, and plant-based protein. Seniors may enjoy the flavorful foods and nutritional advantages of a plant-based diet at lunchtime, including vibrant salads, warming soups, and filling wraps. With lunch options that accommodate a range of tastes and dietary requirements, seniors can easily enjoy the deliciousness of plant-based meals while promoting their health and wellbeing.

CHAPTER 6: FLAVORFUL DINNER RECIPES FOR SENIOR PLANT-BASED EATERS

Seniors have a particular time set aside for dinner where they may have a full meal that feeds both body and spirit. Seniors may choose from a wide array of savory and nutrient-rich plant-based meal alternatives. Let's explore a collection of delectable supper recipes designed for senior plant-based dinners, from warming stews to substantial pasta meals and cuisines from across the world.

1. Rich and creamy coconut lentil curry is made by cooking red lentils with coconut milk, chopped tomatoes, onions, garlic, and curry seasonings. An unique and cozy supper alternative is to serve the curry over brown rice or quinoa and top with fresh cilantro.

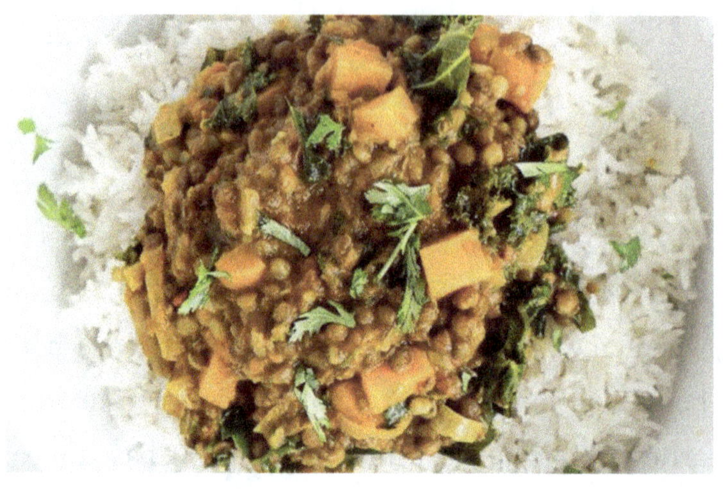

2. Spaghetti with Marinara and vegetarian Meatballs: Make vegan vegetarian meatballs using lentils, mushrooms, oats, and seasonings. For a filling and substantial Italian-inspired supper, top the vegetable meatballs with a tasty marinara sauce and vegan parmesan cheese over whole-grain spaghetti.

3. Roasted Vegetable and Chickpea Quinoa Bowl: Combine chickpeas with a variety of seasonal roasting vegetables, including sweet potatoes, Brussels sprouts, and bell peppers. A vibrant and nutrient-rich supper dish may be made by mixing quinoa with the roasted veggies and chickpeas, then seasoning it with a lemon-tahini sauce.

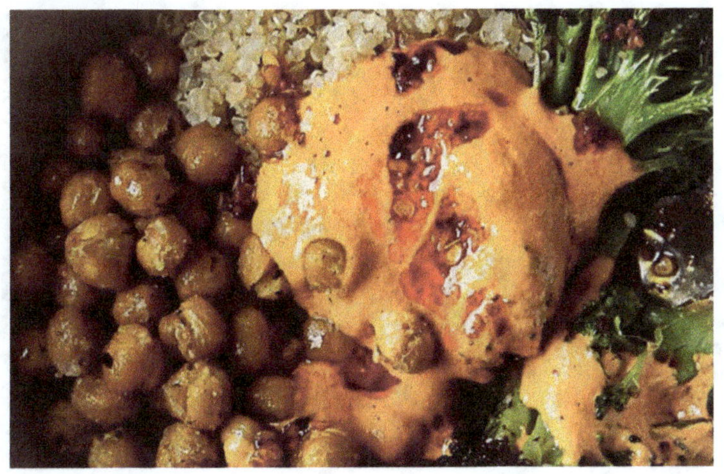

4. Ratatouille with Herbed Quinoa: Create a classic French ratatouille by simmering eggplant, zucchini, tomatoes, and bell peppers in a herb-infused tomato sauce. For a tasty and filling ratatouille meal, serve it over herbed quinoa.

5. Vegan Shepherd's Pie: In a flavorful sauce, combine lentils, carrots, peas, and mushrooms to make a hearty shepherd's pie. A layer of mashed sweet potatoes or cauliflower should be placed on top of the mixture before baking it till golden brown for a filling supper.

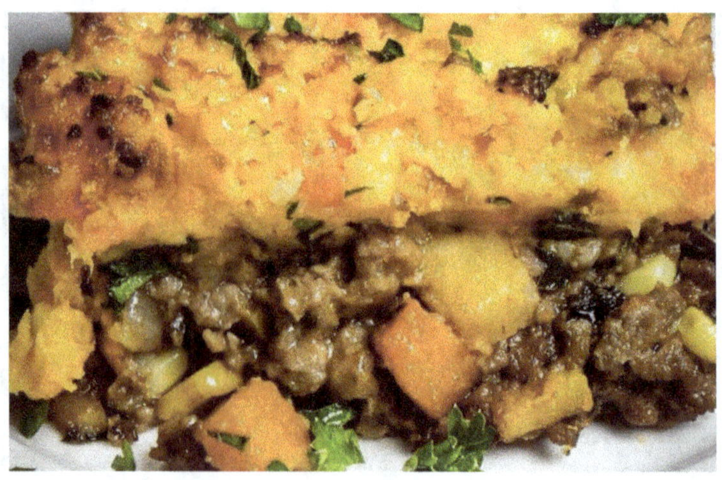

6. Stir-fried veggies with a Thai-inspired sauce consisting of soy sauce, ginger, garlic, and a little sriracha. Included in the mix of bright vegetables are bell peppers, broccoli, carrots, and snow peas. The vegetable stir-fry makes a flavorful and filling supper when served with brown rice or rice noodles.

7. Stuffed Portobello Mushrooms: Place vegan mozzarella, chopped tomatoes, sautéed spinach, and quinoa in big portobello mushrooms. For a gourmet and mouth watering supper, bake the filled mushrooms until they are soft and golden brown.

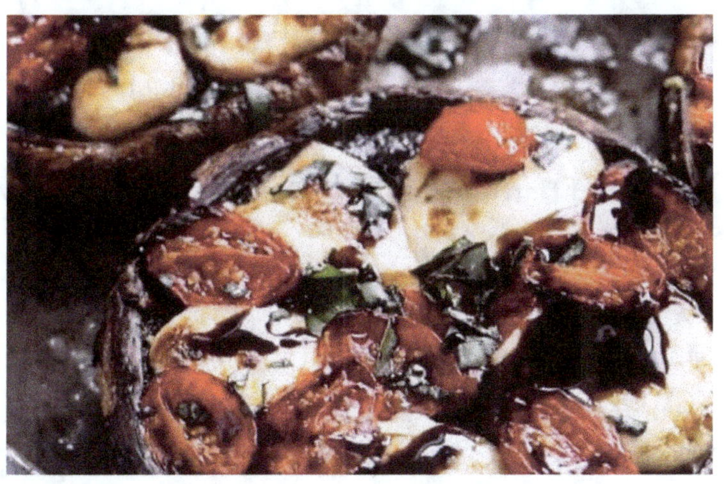

8. Quinoa that has been prepared with black beans, corn, diced tomatoes, avocado, and cilantro is called Mexican-Style Quinoa Salad. A fresh and lively supper with Mexican influences may be made by tossing the quinoa salad with a lime-cumin dressing and serving it over a bed of lettuce or spinach.

9. Vegan Moussaka Inspired by Greek Cuisine: Make a vegan moussaka by layering potatoes, zucchini, and eggplant. Bechamel sauce made from cashews can be drizzled on top. For a delicious and filling supper with a Greek influence, bake the moussaka till bubbling and golden brown.

10. Jackfruit Carnitas Tacos: Jackfruit is simmered with onions, garlic, and Mexican seasonings until it is cooked. Then, the jackfruit is shredded to imitate pulled pork. To give traditional tacos a tasty and vegan twist, serve the jackfruit carnitas in soft corn tortillas with sliced onions, cilantro, and lime wedges.

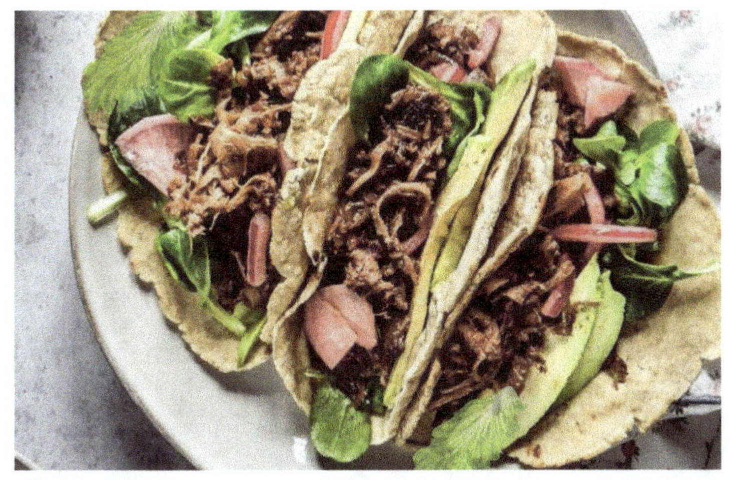

11. Roasted Butternut Squash Risotto: Toss roasted butternut squash with a creamy risotto composed with arborio rice, vegetable broth, and white wine. For a lovely and cozy evening, top the butternut squash risotto with vegan parmesan and sage that has been sliced.

12. Contingent on India Vegetable florets should be marinated in a yogurt-and-Indian-spice combination for the Cauliflower Tikka Masala dish. In a creamy, tomato-based tikka masala sauce, roast the cauliflower until it is caramelized. Enjoy the cauliflower tikka masala for a tasty and fragrant meal together with basmati rice and naan bread.

13. Falafel Wrap with Tahini Sauce: Make falafel by combining chickpeas, spices, and herbs. For a filling and portable supper alternative, serve the falafel in a whole-grain wrap with chopped lettuce, sliced tomatoes, and cucumbers.

14. Hawaiian-Inspired Pineapple Fried Rice: Sautee cooked brown rice with chopped pineapple, bell peppers, carrots, and peas in a Hawaiian-inspired teriyaki sauce. A sweet and delicious meal may be made by topping the pineapple fried rice with chopped scallions, roasted cashews, and sesame seeds.

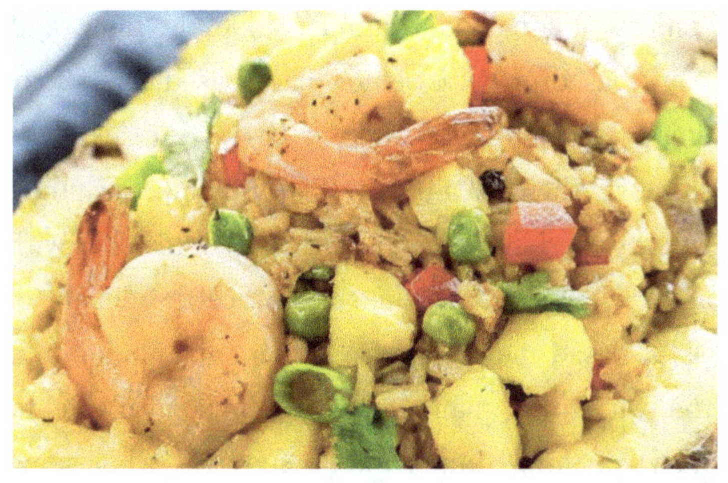

15. Mushroom and Spinach Stroganoff: In a cashew- and nutritional yeast-based creamy stroganoff sauce, saute sliced mushrooms and spinach with onions and garlic. For a hearty and filling meal, serve the mushroom and spinach stroganoff over whole-grain egg noodles.

Finally, plant-based supper ideas for senior diners provide a tantalizing variety of flavours and textures that suit a range of palates and dietary choices. These supper choices provide a broad variety of nutrient-dense plant foods, ensuring that seniors obtain vital vitamins, minerals, fiber, and plant-based protein. Senior plant-based eaters may enjoy scrumptious and satisfying meals that support their health and well-being, including creamy curries, savory pasta dishes, and dishes with a global flair. Seniors may embrace the delight of plant-based meals by using their imagination and the variety of plant-based products available to them, making dinnertime a fun and wholesome part of their daily routine.

CHAPTER 7: SATISFYING PLANT-BASED SNACKS AND APPETIZERS FOR SENIORS

With the chance to indulge in delectable delicacies while preserving health and wellbeing, snacking can be a joyful and fulfilling element of a plant-based lifestyle for seniors. A delicious supplement to any senior's regular eating regimen, plant-based snacks and appetizers are available in a variety of tastes, textures, and nutrients. Let's investigate a few delicious and healthy plant-based snacks and starters that seniors may savor guilt-free:

1. Hummus and Veggie Sticks: This popular and filling plant-based snack combines creamy and savory hummus with vibrant veggie sticks including carrot, cucumber, bell pepper, and celery. The vegetables offer a crisp crunch and an increase in vitamins, while the hummus is a good source of protein, fiber, and other minerals.

2. Guacamole with Whole Grain Tortilla Chips: Guacamole produced from ripe avocados is a delightful and healthy alternative for seniors. It is fresh and creamy. For a nutritious and tasty plant-based snack, serve it with whole grain tortilla chips or baked pita triangles.

3. Nut Butter and Apple Slices: Spreading nut butters like almond, peanut, or cashew over thin slices of crisp apple results in a delicious and satiating snack. It's a delightful option for seniors who want to control their appetite in between meals since it combines fiber, natural sweetness, and healthy fats.

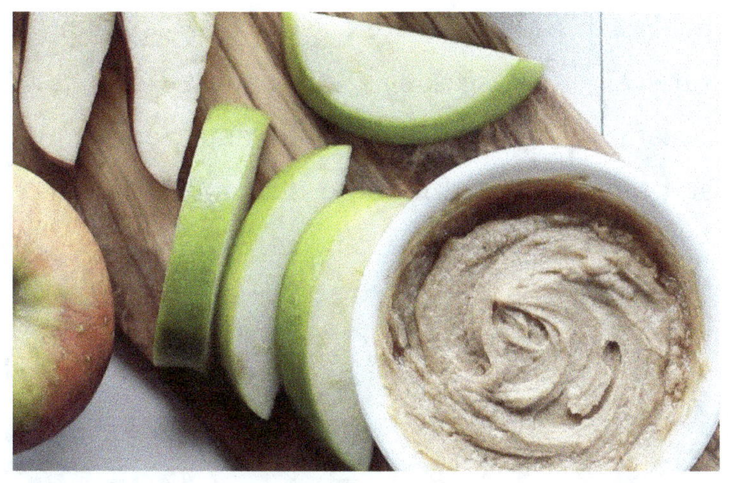

4. Stuffed Bell Peppers: A tasty and filling plant-based snack is made by stuffing roasted bell peppers with a flavorful combination of quinoa, beans, vegetables, and spices. It's a great choice for sharing at events or eating as a light dinner because of its vibrant look and mouth watering tastes.

5. Edamame is a wholesome, high-protein plant food that seniors may enjoy either steamed or roasted. To enhance taste, season with a little sea salt or spice.

6. Fruit Salad: A fruit salad that combines a variety of in-season fruits offers a natural sweetness, vitamins, and antioxidants. Seniors may add their preferred fruits to their fruit salad, such as berries, melon, grapes, and citrus fruits.

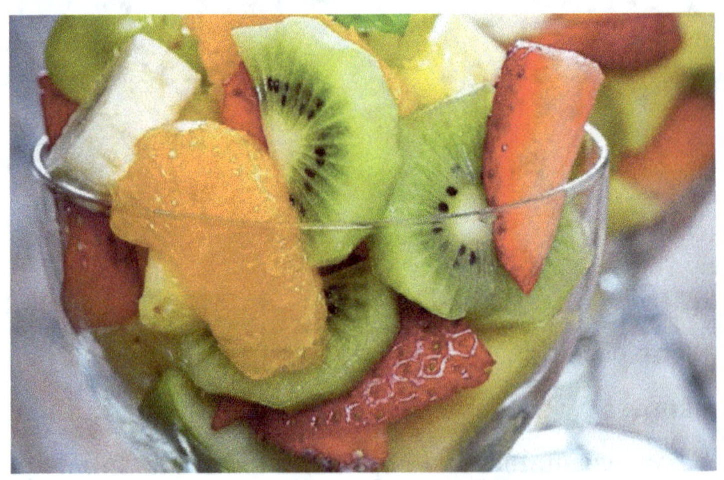

7. Cucumber Avocado Rolls: An exquisite and gratifying plant-based appetizer is made by enclosing creamy avocado in a thin layer of cucumber and finishing it with a dash of salt. These rolls provide a delicious explosion of flavors and a gentle crunch.

8. Roasted Chickpeas: These flavorful, roasted chickpeas are a great plant-based snack for seniors. For a tasty and protein-rich treat, roast them with your preferred spices, such as curry, cumin, or paprika.

9. Vegetable Spring Rolls: An enticing plant-based snack, these savory vegetable spring rolls are loaded with herbs, fresh vegetables, and rice noodles. To enhance the flavor, serve them with a tasty dipping sauce.

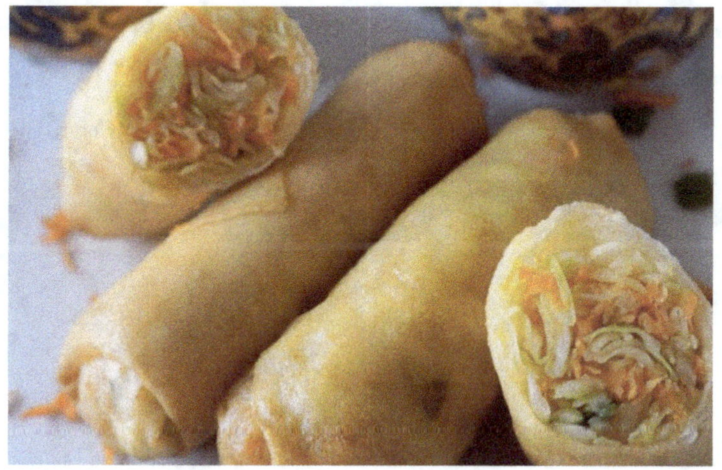

10. Veggie sushi rolls: Avocado, cucumber, and other fresh vegetables are combined to create sushi rolls that are both aesthetically beautiful and fulfilling. With pickled ginger, wasabi, and soy sauce, seniors may savor these rolls.

11. Baked Sweet Potato Fries: Baked sweet potato fries that have been seasoned with herbs and spices provide a pleasant and wholesome plant-based snack option to regular potato chips.

12. Greek Salad Skewers: Threaded on skewers with cherry tomatoes, cucumber, olives, and vegan feta cheese, these tasty and transportable plant-based appetizers are perfect for seniors.

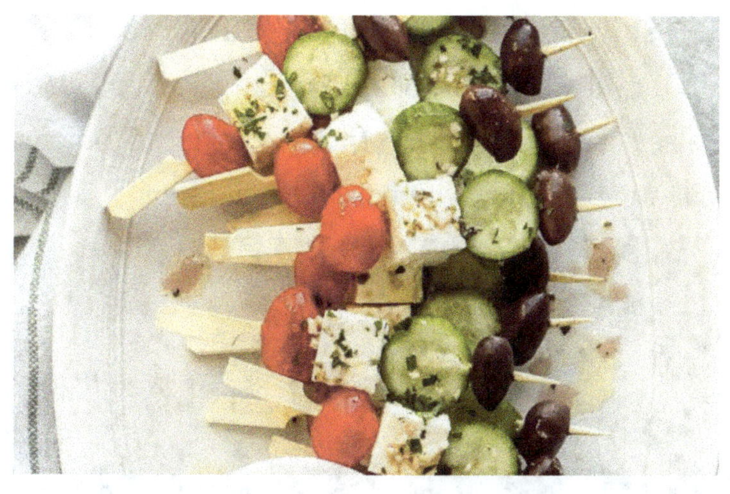

13. Popcorn with nutritional yeast: Air-popped popcorn with a little olive oil drizzle and nutritional yeast on top makes for a flavorful and filling plant-based snack that's high in B vitamins.

14. Rice Paper Rolls: Rice paper rolls stuffed with vibrant vegetables, tempeh or tofu, and fresh herbs provide a tasty and wholesome plant-based appetizer choice.

15. Salsa and Baked Tortilla Chips: For a zesty and guilt-free plant-based snack, mix homemade salsa prepared from fresh tomatoes, onions, cilantro, and lime with baked tortilla chips.

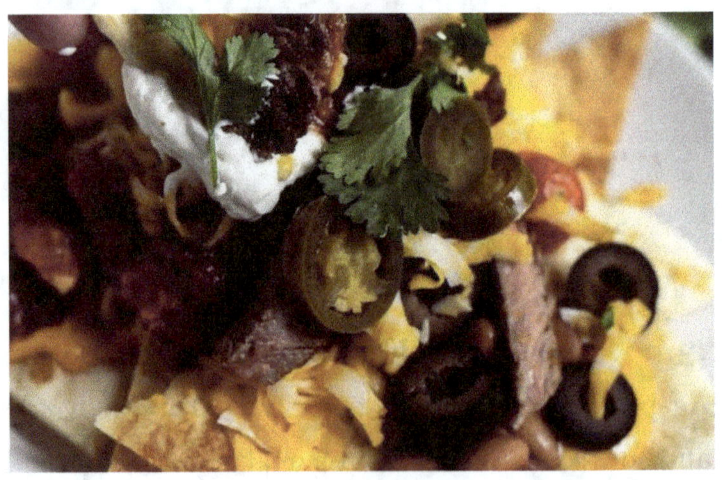

Finally, plant-based snacks and appetizers provide seniors with a variety of tastes and textures to savor while fostering health and wellbeing. These filling and nutrient-dense choices not only tempt the palate, but also provide important vitamins, minerals, and antioxidants. Seniors may indulge in these plant-based snacks and small plates guilt-free in the knowledge that they are providing their bodies with healthful and delicious delicacies. Snacks and appetizers made from plants are guaranteed to be a favorite with seniors looking to adopt a lively and full plant-based lifestyle, whether as a fast pick-me-up or a lovely addition to gatherings.

CHAPTER 8: INDULGENT PLANT-BASED DESSERTS FOR SENIOR SWEET TOOTHS

Who says that if you choose a plant-based diet, you have to give up dessert? There is a wonderful selection of plant-based sweets that are not only tasty but also beneficial for seniors with a sweet craving. Plant-based desserts, which range from rich cakes to creamy puddings, provide a healthier option to conventional sweets while still pleasing even the pickiest senior taste buds. Let's have a look at a wide variety of decadent plant-based sweets that seniors may eat guilt-free.

1. Creamy Vegan Chocolate Mousse: For senior chocolate fans, this velvety, creamy vegan chocolate mousse prepared with avocado, cocoa powder, and maple syrup is a delicious treat. Avocado provides fiber and wholesome fats as well as a velvety texture. For a blast of natural sweetness, garnish with fresh berries.

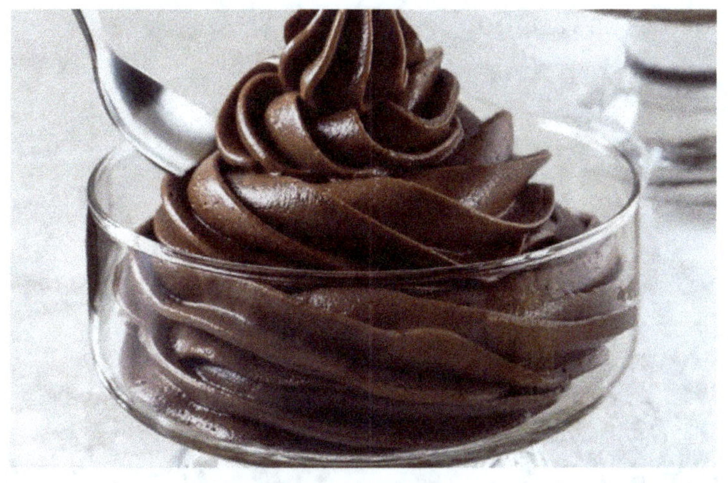

2. Nutty Almond Butter Cups: These delectable plant-based variations on the traditional peanut butter cups are simple to create and full of flavor. These sweets, made with dark chocolate and almond butter, fulfill your hunger for chocolate while giving you a boost of antioxidants and good fats.

3. Rich Vegan Cheesecake: Rich vegan cheesecakes with cashews, coconut cream, and a nutty crust are a show-stopping treat. Add flavors like chocolate, blueberry, or strawberry for a delicious variation.

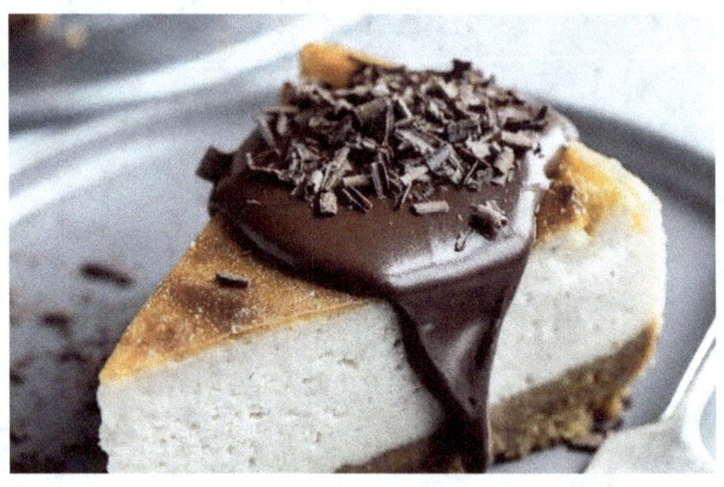

4. Traditional Vegan Brownies: For seniors with a sweet taste, vegan brownies that are chewy and moist are a classic treat. A healthy version of this well-liked treat may be made with ingredients like applesauce, almond flour, and cacao powder.

5. Chia Seed Pudding: A flavor-customizable treat that is filled with nutrients, chia seed pudding may be made in a variety of ways. Chia seeds may be combined with plant-based milk, sweeteners such as maple syrup or agave, and extras like fruits, nuts, or spices for flavor and texture.

6. Nutritious Fruit Crumbles: Fruit crumbles are a soothing and healthy dessert choice for elders. Use a variety of seasonal fruits, such as apples, berries, or peaches, and top with a crumble made of nuts or oats for a pleasant taste contrast.

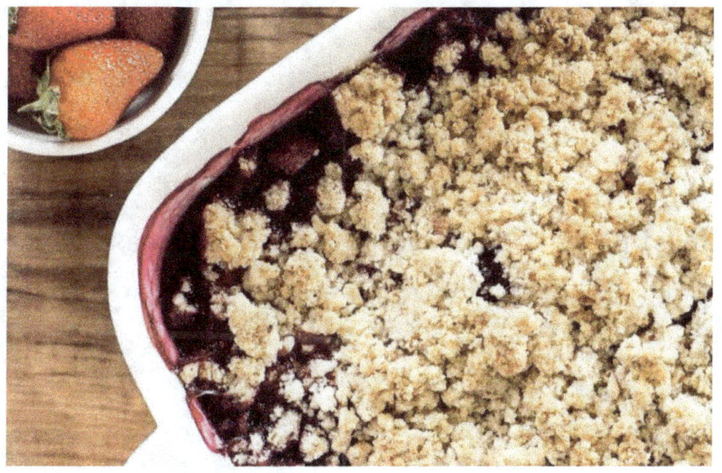

7. Coconut Milk Ice Cream: Ice creams prepared from plant-based milks, such as coconut milk or other plant-based milks, are rich, creamy, and delicious. A wonderful approach to cool yourself on hot days is to choose flavors like chocolate, vanilla, or fruity alternatives.

8. Nutty Energy Balls: Energy balls prepared with nuts, dates, and dried fruit are the ideal on-the-go snack for seniors who lead busy lives. These tasty treats are small enough to eat on the go and are naturally sweetened with sugar.

9. Plant-Based Tiramisu: A sophisticated dessert for seniors to enjoy on special occasions, plant-based tiramisu is constructed with layers of ladyfingers dipped in coffee and rich mascarpone made from cashews.

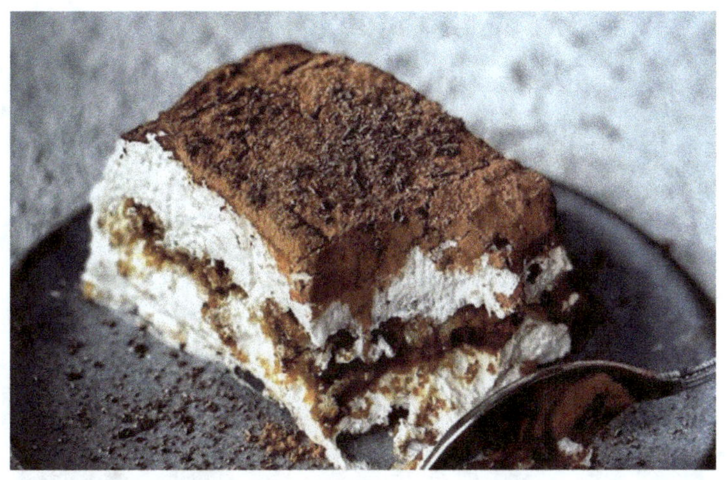

10. Baked Apples with Cinnamon: For a simple yet delectable dessert, serve baked apples with cinnamon sugar and maple syrup on top. Without the extra sugar and bad fats, they provide the cozy and soothing tastes of apple pie.

11. Banana Nice Cream: A tasty and healthful substitute for regular ice cream, banana nice cream is made from pureed bananas. To make a guilt-free frozen dessert, just combine frozen bananas with plant-based milk and flavorings like chocolate or fruit.

12. Vegan Carrot Cake: For seniors who want a traditional cake with a plant-based twist, vegan carrot cake prepared with shredded carrots, almonds, and warming spices is a delectable dessert alternative.

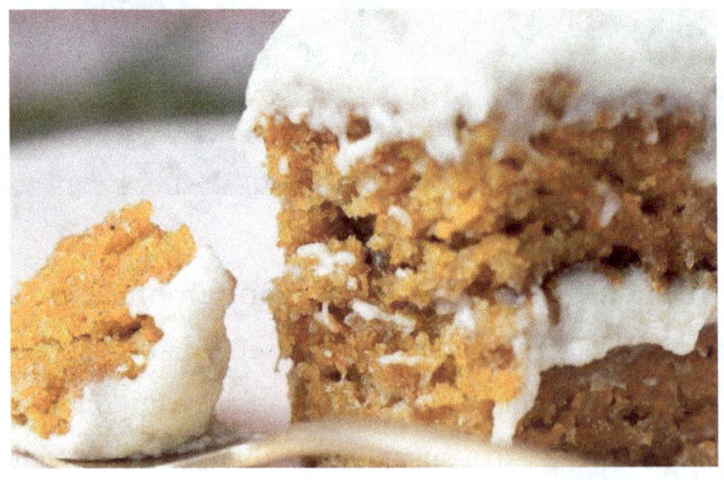

13. Avocado Lime Pie: Avocado lime pie mixes the creamy richness of avocados with the tangy tastes of lime. It is a cool and delicious dessert. Seniors wanting a special and delicious dessert will enjoy this decadent delight.

14. Lemon Poppy Seed Loaf: Made with almond flour, lemon zest, and poppy seeds, lemon poppy seed loaf is a delicious treat for afternoon tea or a fast pick-me-up.

15. Vegan Cinnamon buns: A delicious morning or afternoon treat for seniors with a sweet taste, vegan cinnamon buns are created with healthy wheat flour and plant-based milk. They are soft and cinnamon-spiced.

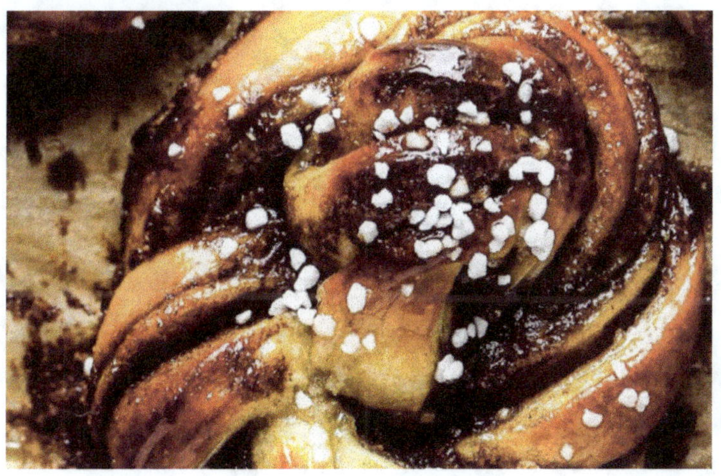

In conclusion, a plant-based diet offers seniors with a sweet craving a variety of decadent dessert options. Plant-based sweets are a delicious way to saute sweet cravings while advancing general health and wellbeing. They range from velvety chocolate mousse to nutritious fruit crumbles and inventive takes on traditional desserts. Knowing that they are sustaining their bodies with nutrient-dense and delectable plant-based foods, seniors may indulge in these treats guilt-free. So go ahead and reward yourself with these decadent plant-based sweets as you enjoy the sweet pleasures of a plant-based diet.

CHAPTER 9: HYDRATING AND NOURISHING PLANT-BASED BEVERAGES FOR SENIORS

Staying hydrated is more crucial as people become older for sustaining overall health and wellbeing. Fatigue, vertigo, and disorientation are just a few of the health problems that may result from dehydration. In addition to offering vital nutrients and fostering hydration, plant-based drinks are an excellent method for seniors to satisfy their thirst. Let's look at some hydrating and filling plant-based drinks that seniors may consume to meet their hydration demands and lead active lives.

1. Herbal teas: Seniors may hydrate and relax with herbal teas such chamomile, peppermint, and ginger. These calming ways to stay hydrated throughout the day may help with digestion, relaxation, and promotion of relaxation.

2. Coconut Water: Coconut water is a natural hydrating elixir that is rich in electrolytes, making it a great choice to replace fluids and important minerals for seniors.

3. Infused Water: By adding energizing tastes to ordinary water, such as lemon, lime, cucumber, or berries, infused water encourages seniors to drink more fluids.

4. Green smoothies: A healthy and hydrating beverage alternative, green smoothies are created with leafy greens, fruits, and plant-based milk. They are abundant in nutrients, vitamins, and antioxidants that promote elder health.

5. Chia Seed Drink: For seniors, chia seed beverages are a hydrating and nutrient-rich choice. Chia seeds have a gel-like consistency that keeps seniors hydrated and satisfied because they absorb water.

6. Watermelon Juice: During the warmer months, seniors may sip on watermelon juice, which is hydrating and refreshing. It is naturally sweet and rich in potassium and vitamin C, among other vitamins and minerals.

7. Almond milk is a delightful plant-based substitute for dairy milk. 7. Seniors may use it as a hydrating beverage on its own or as the foundation for warm beverages or smoothies.

8. Hibiscus Tea: Hibiscus tea provides elders with a vivacious and hydrating choice. Both its refreshing flavor and possible cardiovascular benefits are well-known.

9. Golden Milk: Golden milk, a soothing and hydrating choice for elders, is blended with turmeric, plant-based milk, and warming spices. Anti-inflammatory effects are thought to exist in turmeric.

10. Aloe vera juice: Seniors who choose this hydrated alternative may also benefit from improved intestinal health. It is critical to choose a premium, pure aloe vera juice and use it sparingly.

11. Fruit Infusions: Older adults may make fruit infusions by putting fruit pieces like orange, lemon, or berry slices in a pitcher of water. This enhances their regular hydration regimen with natural sweetness and taste.

12. Papaya Smoothie: A tropical and hydrating beverage choice for seniors is a papaya smoothie blended with plant-based yogurt and a dash of honey. Vitamins and digestive-enhancing enzymes are abundant in papayas.

13. Iced Herbal Lemonade: Iced herbal lemonade mixes lemonade's tartness with the tastes of herbal teas. For hydrating and reviving lemonade variants, seniors might experiment with various herbal tea mixes.

14. Cucumber-mint Water: Seniors may sip on cucumber-mint water throughout the day to stay hydrated and refreshed. It gives simple water a mild taste that is cooling.

15. Carrot-Orange Juice: Carrot-Orange Juice mixes the tangy flavor of oranges with the nutritional advantages of carrots to create a vivacious and hydrating solution. This juice is a good source of beta-carotene and vitamin C.

Finally, plant-based drinks provide seniors with a variety of refreshing and nutritional choices to enhance their health and wellbeing. These plant-based drinks provide older citizens a delectable and delightful way to remain hydrated and fed, ranging from calming herbal teas to nutrient-rich smoothies and refreshing fruit infusions. Seniors may encourage a bright and healthy lifestyle and maintain optimal hydration levels by including these hydrating plant-based drinks into their daily regimen. With these delicious plant-based beverage options, cheers to being hydrated and revitalized!

CHAPTER 10: TIPS FOR DINING OUT AND TRAVELING AS A SENIOR ON A PLANT-BASED DIET

Seniors may find it difficult to follow a plant-based diet while eating out or traveling, but with enough planning and information, it can be a fun and gratifying experience. Here are some helpful suggestions to help seniors maintain their plant-based diet while enjoying excellent meals and experiencing new culinary pleasures, whether you're trying out new eateries or going on a trip.

1. Research Local Restaurants Ahead of Time: Before going out to eat, look up local eateries to see which ones offer plant-based alternatives. Nowadays, many restaurants provide plant-based menus or may accommodate special dietary needs upon request. You may find the top restaurants that welcome plant-based diets by using websites, apps, or online reviews.

2. Call Ahead and Explain Your Needs: If you are confused about the plant-based selections at a restaurant, don't be afraid to call ahead and ask. The personnel will often be happy to meet your demands if you let them know your dietary preferences. To make delectable plant-based meals, chefs might alter recipes or provide suggestions.

3. Examine Ethnic Cuisine: Ethnic eateries, such those serving Mediterranean, Indian, Thai, or Mexican food, often provide a large selection of plant-based meals that are tasty and filling by nature. Take advantage of the chance to experiment with different tastes and cuisines while maintaining your plant-based diet.

4. Emphasize Vegetable-Centric Dishes: Look for recipes that have a lot of vegetables, including salads, stir-fries, vegetable curries, or grain bowls. You can generally customize these choices to make a tasty and wholesome plant-based supper.

5. Build Your Own Meals: Many restaurants provide salad, sandwich, and bowl choices that may be customized. Use this chance to choose plant-based components that suit your dietary choices.

6. When ordering foods that use animal-based products, don't be afraid to inquire about possible substitutes. In place of animal protein, for instance, you might ask for sources of plant-based protein like tofu, tempeh, or beans.

7. Watch Out for Hidden Animal components: Soups, sauces, and dressings may include undetectable animal components. To be sure they are made with plant-based components, inquire about them or order them on the side.

8. Carry Snacks and Plant-Based basics: When traveling, carry plant-based snacks and basics like nuts, seeds, energy bars, or dried fruits.

In situations when there are few other possibilities, these transportable solutions may act as rapid and practical plant-based substitutes.

9. Explore Local Markets and Grocery shops: While traveling, local markets and grocery shops may be a veritable gold mine of plant-based products. To make your meals or snacks, you can get fresh fruits, vegetables, nuts, seeds, and other plant-based ingredients.

10. Examine Plant-Based Travel Destinations: Consider locations recognized for their plant-based food scenes before making trip arrangements. Cities with a wide range of vegan eateries and food trucks might make it easier to go out and discover new cuisines.

11. Take into account hotels with kitchenettes: Whenever feasible, choose lodgings with kitchenettes or access to culinary facilities. This enables you to cook your plant-based meals and take advantage of the freedom of dining at home.

12. Ask for Help from Your Travel Companions: If you're traveling with others, let them know your dietary choices and ask for help in locating plant-based alternatives. They could be willing to explore plant-based cuisine and share fascinating culinary adventures.

13. Embrace Local Produce and Specialties: When eating out or traveling, embrace local food that fits your plant-based diet. Your trip experience may be improved by consuming seasonal fruits, vegetables, and traditional plant-based cuisine.

14. Bring Refillable Water Bottles: It's important to stay hydrated whether traveling or eating out. Bring a reusable water bottle with you so that you can stay hydrated while traveling.

15. Be Flexible and Patient: Keep in mind that traveling and eating out may demand flexibility and patience. Although not all places provide a wide variety of plant-based foods, you may still discover satisfying and fulfilling plant-based meals if you have an open mind and are prepared to investigate.

In conclusion, traveling and eating out as a senior on a plant-based diet can be a joyful journey with careful planning and an adventurous attitude. One may assure a satisfying and gratifying plant-based eating experience by doing restaurant research, articulating your requirements, trying other cuisines, and embracing local vegetables. With these suggestions, seniors may enjoy plant-based meals and make enduring memories while traveling and discovering new culinary treats. Good appetite and safe travels!

Conclusion: Empowering Seniors to Thrive on a Plant-Based Lifestyle

Seniors may thrive in their golden years by adopting a plant-based diet. A plant-based diet offers a plethora of health advantages designed especially for senior well-being thanks to its availability of nutrient-rich fruits, vegetables, whole grains, nuts, seeds, and legumes. The benefits of eating a plant-based diet enable seniors to enjoy active, satisfying lives thanks to healthier immune systems, improved heart health, and better weight control.

Seniors may confidently start their plant-based journey knowing they have the resources to make nutritious decisions thanks to education, awareness, and support. Seniors may enjoy a wide variety of savory plant-based cuisines that are catered to their unique tastes and preferences if they have the knowledge about critical nutrients, imaginative and decadent plant-based meals, and methods for eating out and traveling.

Creating a feeling of community and exchanging stories are other ways to equip elders to flourish on a plant-based diet. Inspiring and motivating one another as they adopt this eating style, seniors may make the path to greater health a group effort. Joining local clubs, attending plant-based events, and making connections with like-minded people may provide helpful tools and a feeling of community on this exciting road.

Furthermore, a plant-based diet has advantages that go beyond general health. Seniors may help make the world a healthier place and leave a good legacy for future generations by adopting eco-friendly and sustainable eating habits.

In conclusion, enabling seniors to flourish on a plant-based diet involves nourishing them on more than just a physical level. It also involves nurturing their spirits, brains, and the environment around them. Seniors have the chance to try other cuisines, enjoy their renewed vigour, and leave a legacy of health and wellbeing. Seniors set out on a journey towards a better, happier, and more rewarding future as they indulge in the nutrition of plant-based foods one that celebrates the delight of flourishing on a plant-based diet.

Appendix A: Shopping List and Pantry Staples for the Senior Plant-Based Cook

For seniors embracing a plant-based lifestyle, having a well-stocked kitchen with essential ingredients is key to creating delicious and nourishing meals. Building a shopping list and keeping a pantry stocked with plant-based staples ensures that seniors can easily whip up a varicty of flavorful dishes. Here's a comprehensive list of shopping items and pantry staples for the senior plant-based cook:

Shopping List:

1. Fresh Fruits:
- Apples
- Bananas
- Berries (strawberries, blueberries, raspberries)
- Citrus fruits (oranges, lemons, limes)
- Avocados
- Grapes
- Melons (watermelon, cantaloupe)
- Kiwi
- Mangoes
- Pears

2. Fresh Vegetables:
- Leafy greens (spinach, kale, arugula, lettuce)
- Broccoli
- Cauliflower
- Carrots
- Bell peppers (assorted colors)
- Tomatoes

- Cucumbers

- Zucchini

- Eggplant

- Sweet potatoes

- Mushrooms

3. Whole Grains:

- Quinoa

- Brown rice

- Farro

- Bulgur

- Whole wheat pasta

- Barley

- Oats (rolled oats or steel-cut oats)

4. Legumes:

- Chickpeas

- Lentils (green, red, or brown)

- Black beans

- Kidney beans

- Cannellini beans

- Pinto beans

5. Nuts and Seeds:
  - Almonds
  - Walnuts
  - Cashews
  - Chia seeds
  - Flaxseeds
  - Pumpkin seeds
  - Sunflower seeds

6. Plant-Based Milk:
  - Almond milk
  - Soy milk
  - Oat milk
  - Coconut milk (canned or carton)

7. Tofu and Tempeh:
  - Firm tofu
  - Silken tofu
  - Tempeh

8. Plant-Based Yogurt:

- Almond yogurt

- Coconut yogurt

- Soy yogurt

9. Plant-Based Protein:

- Plant-based burgers or sausages

- Seitan

- Plant-based protein powder (optional for smoothies)

10. Herbs and Spices:

- Basil

- Oregano

- Thyme

- Rosemary

- Cumin

- Paprika

- Turmeric

- Ginger

- Garlic powder

- Onion powder

- Cinnamon

- Nutmeg

11. Condiments and Sauces:

- Extra virgin olive oil

- Balsamic vinegar

- Soy sauce (or tamari for gluten-free option)

- Tahini

- Mustard

- Hot sauce

- Salsa

- Tomato sauce (check for no added sugars)

12. Sweeteners:

- Maple syrup

- Agave nectar

- Coconut sugar

- Date syrup

13. Miscellaneous:

- Vegetable broth (low-sodium)

- Nutritional yeast

- Baking essentials (baking powder, baking soda)

Pantry Staples:

1. Dried fruits:
  - Raisins
  - Apricots
  - Dates

2. Whole Grain Flours:
  - Whole wheat flour
  - Almond flour
  - Coconut flour

3. Plant-Based Butter or Margarine

4. Canned Goods:
  - Diced tomatoes
  - Tomato paste
  - Coconut cream
  - Unsweetened applesauce

5. Canned Beans:
  - Chickpeas
  - Black beans

- Kidney beans

6. Dried Pasta (whole wheat or gluten-free)

7. Whole Grain Crackers or Rice Cakes

8. Herbal Teas

9. Dried Herbs and Spices:
  - Basil
  - Oregano
  - Thyme
  - Rosemary
  - Cumin
  - Paprika
  - Turmeric
  - Ginger
  - Garlic powder
  - Onion powder
  - Cinnamon
  - Nutmeg

10. Nondairy Sweeteners:

- Stevia (if preferred)

The senior plant-based chef may make a broad range of tasty, wholesome, and fulfilling meals by having these ingredients on hand. Seniors may easily take advantage of the health advantages and gastronomic joys of a plant-based diet if they keep their pantries well-stocked and regularly buy for fresh vegetables at the grocery store.

Appendix B: Frequently Asked Questions about Plant-Based Eating for Seniors

1. Is a plant-based diet appropriate for older citizens?

Yes, elders may benefit from a plant-based diet. It offers necessary vitamins, minerals, antioxidants, and fiber that promote heart health, brain function, and general wellbeing. An optimally balanced plant-based diet may benefit seniors.

2. Will a plant-based diet provide me with adequate protein?

■Yes, plant-based foods including legumes, tofu, tempeh, nuts, seeds, and healthy grains may provide seniors with enough protein. A sufficient intake of protein is ensured by include a range of these foods in meals.

3. Can an elderly person maintain their weight better on a plant-based diet?

■Yes, weight management may benefit from a plant-based diet that prioritizes whole foods and limits processed foods. It usually has less calories and saturated fats, which supports maintaining a healthy weight.

4. What are some simple vegan dishes for older people?

■Simple plant-based dishes like vegetable stir-fries, bean-based salads, fruit and vegetable smoothies, vegetable soups, and grain bowls with a variety of toppings are perfect for seniors.

5. How can I make sure that a plant-based diet gives me adequate nutrients?

To get different nutrients, one must eat a variety of plant-based meals. After speaking with a healthcare provider, seniors may also want to think about taking vitamin B12 and vitamin D supplements if they're in need of them.

6. Can a vegan diet help my heart health as I become older?

Yes, a plant-based diet may improve heart health by lowering blood pressure and cholesterol levels. It contains plenty of fiber, potassium, and antioxidants, all of which are good for the heart.

7. Is eating a plant-based diet expensive?

Budget-friendly plant-based diets are possible, particularly when they emphasize whole foods like grains, legumes, and locally available veggies. Seniors may save money by planning their meals and buying in bulk.

8. Can a plant-based diet aid elders with digestive problems?

Yes, the fiber included in plant-based diets may assist regular bowel motions and help with digestion. Seniors with particular digestive problems should speak with a healthcare provider for individualized guidance.

9. How can someone who follows a plant-based diet manage social settings and eating out?

Seniors may inform hosts or restaurants in advance of their dietary preferences in social circumstances. To make sure they have adequate alternatives, they might also offer to bring a food that is made of plants to meetings.

10. Will eating a plant-based diet make me feel younger and more lively as I become older?

Many seniors who eat a plant-based diet say it has given them more energy and vigor. Consuming meals that are high in nutrients may improve overall health and promote an active lifestyle.

11. Is it possible to manage chronic medical illnesses with a plant-based diet?

Adopting a plant-based diet may help you manage illnesses like type 2 diabetes and hypertension that are chronic. However, seniors should collaborate with their medical professionals to customize their diet to their unique medical requirements.

12. Is it difficult to discover plant-based choices while dining out or traveling?

Nowadays, because to more availability and knowledge, it might be simpler to find plant-based choices whether traveling or eating out. There are often more plant-based options when researching restaurants beforehand or while exploring regional cuisines.

13. Can a senior who follows a plant-based diet indulge in rich sweets and treats?

The answer is that seniors may enjoy a broad range of sweets and snacks produced from plant-based components such fruits, nuts, and plant-based milk. To satiate a sweet need, there are many inventive dishes available.

14. As a senior, how can I make sure I get adequate calcium on a plant-based diet?

Seniors may get calcium through plant-based foods including almonds, tofu, fortified plant milks, and leafy greens. Having a well-rounded, diversified diet can assist assure getting enough calcium.

15. Can an elderly person's brain health and cognitive performance be improved by a plant-based diet?

Undoubtedly, a plant-based diet high in antioxidants and good fats may promote brain function and perhaps reduce the incidence of cognitive decline in older people.

Finally, adopting a plant-based diet as an elderly person might bring up a number of concerns, but with the correct knowledge and direction, seniors can confidently take advantage of the health advantages and gastronomic joys of plant-based eating. As usual, seeking tailored guidance from a medical expert or registered dietician may help seniors succeed in their plant-based journey.

Appendix C: Additional Resources for Seniors Interested in a Plant-Based Lifestyle

1. Books:

"How Not to Die" by Dr. Michael Greger

"The Blue Zones Kitchen" by Dan Buettner

"Forks Over Knives: The Plant-Based Way to Health" by Gene Stone and T. Colin Campbell

"The Plant-Based Solution" by Joel K. Kahn, MD

"The Longevity Diet" by Valter Longo

2. Websites and Blogs:

Nutritionfacts.org: Provides evidence-based information on plant-based nutrition and health.

Forks Over Knives: Offers plant-based recipes, meal plans, and success stories.

Oh She Glows: A popular plant-based food blog with a variety of delicious recipes.

■Plant-Based Cooking: A resource for plant-based recipes and cooking tips for seniors.

3. Apps:

■Forks Over Knives: Offers plant-based recipes and meal planning tools.

■HappyCow: Helps seniors find plant-based restaurants and vegan-friendly options while traveling.

■Daily Dozen: Developed by Dr. Michael Greger, this app helps track daily servings of plant-based foods.

4. Online Courses and Webinars:

■Plant-Based Nutrition Certificate: Offered by eCornell in collaboration with T. Colin Campbell Center for Nutrition Studies.

■Physicians Committee for Responsible Medicine (PCRM) webinars: Covers various aspects of plant-based nutrition and health.

5. YouTube Channels:

■Nutritionfacts.org: Features informative videos on plant-based nutrition and health by Dr. Michael Greger.

■The Happy Pear: Offers fun and easy plant-based recipe videos.

■Sweet Potato Soul: Provides delicious and creative plant-based recipes.

6. Social Media:

■Instagram: Follow plant-based influencers, chefs, and nutritionists for inspiration and recipe ideas.

■Facebook Groups: Join plant-based and vegan communities to connect with like-minded individuals and share experiences.

7. Local Support:

■Check for local plant-based or vegan meetups in the area. Seniors can attend events, workshops, or cooking classes to connect with others on the same journey.

8. Dietitian Consultation:

■Consider consulting with a registered dietitian or nutritionist who specializes in plant-based nutrition. They can provide personalized advice and address specific concerns.

9. Senior Centers and Community Programs:

■Inquire if local senior centers or community programs offer plant-based cooking classes or workshops.

10. Documentaries:

- "Forks Over Knives": An informative documentary advocating for the health benefits of a plant-based diet.
- "Game Changers": Explores the performance benefits of a plant-based diet for athletes.
- "What the Health": Investigates the impact of animal-based foods on health.

Remember that every individual's journey to a plant-based lifestyle is unique, and it's essential for seniors to explore resources that align with their specific preferences and health needs. With the wealth of information available, seniors can confidently embark on their plant-based journey and enjoy the health benefits and culinary delights of this vibrant lifestyle.

"Uncover the benefits of a plant-based diet! Thrive with our senior-friendly cookbook. Enjoy wonderful meals today and embrace health!" Simply Add To Cart!!!